WEIGHT LOSS FOR WOMEN OVER 50:

THE ULTIMATE GUIDE TO TRANSFORM YOUR MIND & BODY FOREVER

Introduction

I want to thank you and congratulate you for downloading the book "Weight Loss for Women Over 50: The Ultimate Guide to Transform Your Mind & Body Forever."

The road to health and fitness over the age of 50 comes with its own unique set of challenges, but it is by no means impossible. There is clearly a lot of confusion and frustration surrounding this topic, but hopefully this book will shed some much needed light on it, and become a guide that you can refer to when you may hit a roadblock or hurdle in your journey to weight loss and fitness.

Society tells us that we lose value as we age. Especially for women, this can be a devastating occurrence. But we don't have to accept this fate. There are many women in their 50's, 60's and beyond who are disproving the myth that your value ends once you are over the age of 50. They are fit, healthy and making large contributions to the world.

There are many things that hinder us in life from achieving our goals, but the main thing is ourselves. Anything is possible if you have the desire, drive and determination to make it happen. You are the architect of your life and only you can make the change you want. I hope that you reach all of your fitness goals regardless of what age you are right now. I hope this is only the beginning.

Chapter 1

Challenges losing weight after 50

So as most of you already know, losing weight and keeping it off after the age of 50 has its challenges. In fact, 70% of people over 50 are overweight in the US. One third of those are classified as obese. Complications from these issues cost us 190 billion dollars a year to treat. Obesity also shortens the life span. Studies show that obese people live 3-10 years less than their average weight counterparts. This is the same loss of life span that smokers experience. In fact more than 80% of Type 2 diabetes is linked to weight. In addition, one in three cancer deaths is linked to poor nutrition, no physical activity, and excess body weight. These are very scary statistics, but hope is not lost, you can turn it around, engage in healthy habits, and sustain a healthy weight.

It does become more difficult to sustain weight as we age, but it is definitely possible and definitely doable. There are several key factors that contribute to the body holding onto more weight as we age, including: reduced metabolism, increased hunger, not getting enough sleep, loss of muscle mass. Let's examine these one by one.

Reduced Metabolism

First, let's take a look at reduced metabolism. I'm sure you remember the days when you could eat a burger and fries and dessert and have nothing to worry about weight wise. Now, it seems that the day after you eat a couple of donuts, you've gained 5 pounds. This is because your metabolism slows down 5 percent every decade after age 40. Your metabolism is the mechanism your body uses to convert food into energy. So when it's not working like it used to, your body doesn't burn calories the way it used to, and the result is you guessed it: you gain weight much more easily. Many experts say that to counteract this, you should consume approximately 100 fewer calories per day than you normally would (if you are in a weight maintenance mode, not weight loss mode). It's not actually terribly hard to do, you just have to pay attention to creamy salad dressings and think about the extra cheese or mayo that you may be used to putting on sandwiches. If you switch to balsamic dressings (or oil and vinegar), or skip the full fat mayo for a lower calorie condiment, you should be fine. It's an easy strategy to cut out the 100 calories per day without having to think about it too much.

Increased Hunger

No you weren't imagining it, you are feeling hungrier. After 40, your estrogen levels decline sharply, and as a result, your thyroid and blood sugar are affected. This causes you to become hungrier, and gain weight if you're not careful. This in combination with the loss of muscle mass (since muscle burns fat), means that again, you're burning fewer calories.

You may not have any control over your hormone levels, but you can counteract some of the damage by changing some things in your diet. For example, switch from the empty calories of junk food for foods with more fiber. Fiber not only is great for keeping your digestive system regular and functioning well, but it helps you feel fuller faster and longer. Foods that contain a good amount of fiber to keep you full include:

Beans

Berries

Air popped popcorn

Wild rice

Peas

Spinach

Greens

Nuts

Squash

Potatoes

Bananas

Apples

There are many others as well, but these should get you started.

Not getting enough sleep

I understand completed, you have a high stress job, or kids to take to school or x,y,z going on with no time to get enough rest. It's completely understandable. The high stress is also probably the reason why you reach for a donut or muffin instead of a healthy breakfast or don't feel like working out because you ate a fast food for lunch. We've all been there.

The issue is that sleeps helps you lose weight, and not getting enough of it consistently will definitely help you gain weight. Many studies have studied the link between sleep and weight, and in one study it showed that not getting enough sleep actually makes you crave sugary high calorie foods!

The best to aim for if you are not getting the sleep you need is 7.5 -8.5 hours a night. If you're getting significantly less than that, you must try to get the recommended amount you need. You may need to participate in a sleep study to figure out why you're not sleeping, it could be due to any number of issues including sleep apnea or insomnia.

Loss of muscle mass

As we age, we naturally lose muscle mass, and since muscles burn 3 x more calories than fat does, you can see why many of us gain weight after 50. In addition, testosterone levels drops with age as well as estrogen, and if muscles aren't being used or strengthened during this time, you will lose them.

The good news is you can counteract this. By engaging in regular strength training, you will increase your metabolism and burn more calories daily. For each pound of muscle you build, you will burn 50 calories per day at rest. Meaning, if you build 10 lbs of muscle that's a whopping 500 calories per day that you'll burn! In addition, building muscle can also protect bones and help prevent osteoporosis.

Chapter 2

Nutrition for weight loss after 50

So now that we know the hurdles that we have to overcome to get the weight off and keep it off, let's get started on the game plan for how to actually make it happen. We're going to address what you should be eating, how much and in what portions you should be eating and when you should be eating for optimal weight loss.

What to eat

Once we reach our 50's every calorie counts, and it's necessary to make sure the foods you eat are helping you on your weight loss journey and not hindering you. This is why you should embrace eating a whole food, primal style diet. This means for the majority of your meals you should be eating foods that contain minimal additives. Try to stay far far away from processed foods. Eat humanely raised animal proteins, or if you're vegetarian, eat lots of protein rich foods such as beans, peas, chickpeas, quinoa or seitan. In addition, you should be eating fresh vegetables and fruits with most meals as well. You should also eat low fat dairy foods such as low fat cheese, yogurt and cottage cheese. Generally decreasing your consumption of high fructose corn syrup, sugar etc. will not only benefit your overall health, but will help you shed the pounds more quickly.

In addition, if you are gluten free, don't think that gluten free products are all good. Many gluten free products substitute a lot of the starch in the form of potato and other types of flours. In that case, you're just substituting one high blood sugar spike for another.

In fact AARP (American Association of Retired Persons) a US based membership and interest group for people age 50 and older, has come up with a recommended healthy eating plan, specifically for those in the 50 plus age group. They worked with NIH (National Institutes of Health) to study the correlation between lifestyle choices and cancer as well as other diseases among those 50 and older.

They came up with a healthy eating plan called the New American Diet. It contains healthy eating tips and recommendations that will lead to better health and wellness as well as weight loss. It's less like a traditional diet and more like a new way of relating to food. The key is you have to commit to make a lifestyle change, and stick to it long-term, so you should find an eating plan that makes it easy for you to stick with. Their plan is good because it gives you basic principles to work with instead of rigid rules, and recommends eating whole foods which we should all be doing anyway.

The AARP plan is detailed below:

1. Eat breakfast every day-Eating breakfast each day is a great way to rev up your metabolism and help get you started for the day's tasks. Eat a breakfast full of protein, whole grains and fruit. It will keep your insulin levels high and keep you from overeating later in the day.

2. Eat lots of fruit and vegetables- This one I know you've heard before, but it really is true. Some diets discourage you from eating fruit, but eating fruit not only helps you lose weight but can also help you live longer as well. Not to mention, fruits are high in antioxidants, which fight free radicals in the body and prevent cell damage.

3. Drink more water- Many times you may not realize how many calories you are consuming through what you drink. We drink soda, juice, alcohol, and other beverages throughout the day and that can really add a lot of calories. Drinking sodas, even diet soda increases the body's cravings for sweet high calorie foods.

4. Eat more fish- Fish is a key component in AARP's eating plan. It has the omega 3 fatty acids that your body needs for brain health, and is low in calories. The omega 3's in fish may lower your risk for particular cancers and help lessen the effects of certain inflammatory diseases such as rheumatoid arthritis. On the other end of the spectrum eating hot dogs and

sausages has been shown to have the opposite effect, so it's recommended to not eat them frequently.

5. Love whole grain-Whole grains are a fantastic source of vitamins but also fiber. The AARP/NIH study shows that regularly eating whole grain bread, whole wheat pasta and brown rice can lessen your risk of heart disease, respiratory illness, and some cancers including colon and breast cancers. In addition, whole grains help you lose weight, in particular belly fat.

6. Inspect food labels-Women who regularly read food labels are on average 9 pounds lighter than women who don't. Just choose foods that are lower in sugar and calories in general, and high in nutrients and you should be fine.

7. Dine in not out for 2 weeks- Dining out carries a lot of potential risks. You don't know exactly how the food was made, or what specific ingredients were added to sauces, etc. Not to mention the fact that on average restaurant meals are 2-3 times larger than the recommended serving sizes. For reference, fruits and vegetables should be the size of your fist, meat should be no bigger than a deck of cards, and fish should be about the size of a checkbook.

8. Snack during the day- The data shows that people who snack twice a day lose more weight than those who only eat 3 large meals per day. One snack between breakfast

and lunch, the other between lunch and dinner. Snacks should consist of healthy foods such as nuts, fruit or veggies with hummus or peanut butter, or a simple fruit such as an apple or pear.

9. Chew gum- I couldn't believe this one either. Chewing gum releases hormones that tell your brain that you're full. It also helps if you're like me and like to snack haphazardly while watching TV, cooking or you name it. Just remember always choose sugar free, sugar filled gum will hurt your teeth and cause tooth decay.

Ghrelin

Another thing to consider is the existence of Ghrelin. For those of you who have never heard of it, let me explain. Ghrelin is a hormone that controls hunger and drives your appetite. If you don't understand Ghrelin, how it works and how to control it, you can forget about losing weight. It is a survival hormone that is secreted in the stomach that ensures that we eat. Research shows that it spikes when we skip meals, after exercise, when dieting, lack of sleep and when avoiding carbs. In order to keep Ghrelin under control:

1. Don't skip meals-You must eat every 3-4 hours to control Ghrelin, depending on how long you stay awake during a normal day, that may mean 4-6 meals and snacks.

2. Eat breakfast within an hour of waking up- It is the most crucial meal of the day. It will determine how much you will eat at 3 pm. Eat soon upon waking and take control of Ghrelin.

3. Try to keep a balance of protein and carbs at each meal or snack- You get the best combination of nutrients to fight hunger and cravings, and feel full. Protein increases your metabolism while carbs keep your Ghrelin in check and stimulate brain functioning.

4. Follow the 70/30 rule- The 70/30 rule states that you should eat 70% of your food for the day before dinner and only 30% at dinner. Also ensure you eat dinner at least 90 minutes before (but preferably 2-3 hours) you go to sleep so that you can sleep well.
5. Drink water- I know I said it once, but I'll say it again for good measure. It's essential for keeping metabolism going strong, burning fat and keeping energy high.

Chapter 3

Exercise for optimal weight loss after 50

Since we know that we lose muscle mass after 50, the goal is to boost our muscle mass consistently and make regular exercise part of daily and weekly life. The best way to get started is to get familiar with weight training, but the ultimate goal is to find the form of exercise that you truly love (or at least don't hate, and stick with it). It's best to find your primary cardio exercise that you like and then add your weight training into the mix. So if you love running great, go with that, if you hate it, find something else. Maybe it's spinning, or maybe it's the elliptical machine, or hip hop dance class. It's just whatever you love to do, find it, and continue to do it.

In terms of your weight training, here are a few helpful tips to get you started.

How much weight to use?

Figuring out how much weight you should use depends on the number of repetitions you can do successfully. Ideally, you want to lift weight that you can properly do for 8-15 reps. It is suggested that you build up the number of reps to 20 or so, and then once you get comfortable at that weight, add additional weight until you are comfortable at 20 reps and so on.

How many reps and sets are optimal?

Traditionally when weight training for strength, you should aim for three to five sets of 8 to 12 reps. But that may be too high of a goal, due to increased joint injury in older people, so a better idea is to mix it up somewhat in terms of reps. So instead of three sets of pure bicep curls, you can do a set or two of pulldowns or tricep work, and then a set of bicep curls and include a squat or lunge. Of course do what works best for you, so if you want to do your reps straight, by all means go for it!

How often should you do weight training?

In the beginning, and especially if you're new to weight training you will benefit from doing twice per week weight training sessions. Each session should last 20-30 minutes and you should be working one main body area each session. So during one session you could focus on arms, then the next session should focus on legs, etc.

Once you are comfortable with the two day weight training schedule you should increase it to 3-4 times per week. Just remember that weight training usually requires a day of rest from weights for that body area, so if you focus on legs one day, then don't turn around and do legs again the next day, although you can do cardio the following day.

How do you know when it's time to increase the resistance?

It depends mainly on you, but once you can lift a weight 15-20 times without pain it's time to add more resistance or more weight. It's recommended that you add resistance to larger muscle groups such as legs 10% at a time, and for smaller muscle groups such as arms 5% at a time. So if you are currently using 100 pounds for your legs, you could add 10 lbs. at a time, but for your arms only add 5.

What type of weights should you use?

In terms of weights, there are many different types to choose from including: kettle bells, tubing, dumbbells among others. The key is to choose the right type for you that you feel comfortable controlling and that is appropriate for the muscle group that you're working on. For example a dumbbell chest press-lying on your back pushing weights overhead-works the same muscle groups as a tubing exercise where you have the tubing latched to a door and are pressing handles towards the center. The exercise using the tubing may be easier for beginners to complete.

Also, always remember to stretch your muscles after they are warmed up or in other words at the end of your weight workout. I know it may seem counterintuitive, but stretching the muscle before you workout can cause a variety of problems. First, it may cause a loss of strength during your lifting and training time, and it may even cause minor strains or worse muscle tears.

Cardio

Next let's look at some cardiovascular exercise that you should be doing as well which strengthens your heart, increases your recovery time, and helps increase metabolism.

Ideally, you should be doing some sort of exercise 4-5 times per week, mixing cardio in either before your weight training workout, or on alternating days if you prefer.

In order to lose weight most effectively, I recommend doing an interval training program for your cardio routine. If you are not familiar with interval training , it's pretty simple. Interval training is when you alternate speed or intensity throughout your workout for improved effectiveness. For example, you may start out running full speed for 2 minutes, then slow down a light jog for 1 minute, then return to a full run for 2 minutes etc. Interval training has been shown to have significant benefits over straight slow cardio workouts, because you will burn more calories throughout the day due to the afterburner effect. The other added benefit is that your workouts are going to be shorter than your slow go cardio routine. So what's not to love about that! Here are a few sample interval workouts for you to try.

Outdoor walking interval routine

This is one of the simplest interval routines there is. You can also customize it by starting out with equal walk and jog times, and then increase the run or jog times once you're ready.

Walk 2 minutes

Jog/run 1 minute

Walk 2 minutes

Jog/run 1-1/2 minutes

Walk 1 minute

Jog/run 2 minutes

Walk 2 minutes

Jog/run 1-1/2 minute

Walk 1 minute

Jog/run 2 minutes

Elliptical training

Initially, you should be spending more time in the low interval than in the high interval. Then gradually even it out so that you're spending equal amounts of time in the high and the low. Eventually once you get used to it, you should be spending more time at your high intensity level.

Low resistance for 90 seconds

High resistance for 30 seconds

Low resistance for 90 seconds

High resistance for 45 seconds

Low resistance for 90 seconds

High resistance for 30 seconds

Low resistance for 90 seconds

High resistance for 45 seconds

Treadmill interval training

For this plan, you should warm up with a steady walking pace for 5 minutes and then:

30 seconds fast, 30 seconds slow

45 seconds fast, 45 seconds slow

60 seconds fast, 60 seconds slow

90 seconds fast, 90 seconds slow

60 seconds fast, 60 seconds slow

45 seconds fast, 45 seconds slow

30 seconds fast, 30 seconds slow

Keep in mind to stop if you start to feel pain or feel otherwise unable to continue. Also please consult your doctor before starting any new diet or exercise plan.

Chapter 4

Mental Strength for Weight Loss Success

I know that if you're anything like me, you have tried a thousand diet and just as many exercise programs before, with varying degrees of success. In our stressful society where things are getting increasingly more complicated every day, it is a definite challenge to not only lose weight, but keep the weight off. The people that are successful know that it takes more than just diet and exercise to get and stay fit. It takes mental toughness and determination, and the willpower to say no to things you know are terrible for your health and future. This is not to say that you can't indulge your sweet tooth now and then, or you can't enjoy a rich meal occasionally, it just means on the day to day, meaning most days, you will need to commit to your new life choice to become healthy and lose weight. I am including some techniques that helped me lose 40 pounds three years ago and keep it off to this day. It hasn't always been easy, but if I can do it, so can you. Trust me, I was a junk food junkie who loved chips, cookies, cake, chocolate you name it, and I probably had a stash somewhere. But I knew I had to make some serious changes and I dedicated myself to that goal.

I have included some strategies and tips to help you develop the mental beliefs and attitudes you need to cultivate in order to become successful.

Self talk

The best way to turn around any of the blocks that have been stopping you from reaching your goals, is having great self talk. This will help you change your core thoughts and beliefs about diet and exercise.

In order to get the most out of any diet and exercise program, you have to reprogram your mind to get aligned with your goals. Here are some keys changes that you should need to make in order to ensure your success.

1. Don't view dieting as drudgery that you can only do for short periods of time. Instead look at dieting as a strategy to keep you healthy, looking good and feeling great.
2. Don't look at exercise as an added burden on your life. People who are in shape see exercise as a mandatory habit for physical and mental health and wellness. Regardless of how many hours you work, or how many children you have or whatever your responsibilities are, you must make exercise a part of your life on a regular basis.
3. Expect to have cravings and times when you want to stray from your diet and exercise plan. You should have

a plan in place to overcome it and stay compliant with your diet.

Negative: Dieting equals pain

Positive: Dieting equals pleasure through feeling successful, having more energy, and happy with my body.

Negative: Diets don't work.

Positive: My diet works perfectly every time, as long as I follow it.

Negative: Dieting means denying myself pleasure.

Positive: Dieting creates the power of being fit, healthy and looking my best.

Negative: Dieting is too much work.

Positive: Being overweight is too much work.

Here are some exercises to help you even more.

Exercises

Write down why you weren't successful in your past attempt to lose weight

Did you lack the motivation, time, plan? What was the reason?

Next, write down all the negative things in your life now, that are related to your weight?

Write down what your life will be like if you don't lose the weight and keep doing what you're doing.

What things will you miss out on?

Write down your three month, six month, and year goals? Where do you want to be fitness wise?

Be realistic about your goals. You should use a 2 lb. per week average weight loss as your goal.

Write your goals down and place them somewhere where you will see them regularly on a daily basis. While you're exercising, visualize your success. See your healthier, slimmer self in your mind's eye. Feel what it will feel like to be at your goal weight. Act as if you have already reached your goals. When a situation arises that can throw you off track from your goal, like the cake or donuts at work, or not working out for a week, think about the fit you would act, and do what they would do, which is stick to the plan.

Also, you may want to come up with a positive affirmation to say to yourself to help keep you motivated while you are working out, or to keep you from straying from your diet.

I have added some samples below:

My health is improving and so is my life.

Every day I am feeling healthier and stronger.

Every day and in every way I am getting slimmer and fitter.

I love eating healthy food and it helps me reach my ideal weight.

I love exercising daily and it helps me reach my ideal weight.

The idea is just memorize one or two of these affirmations so that if you are feeling off kilter in any way with your plan, you can have something that bolsters you and reminds you why you're doing it.

Chapter 5

Inspiration

I am a big advocate of the theory that seeing is believing. If you see for yourself some examples of women who are over 50, fit and fabulous they can act as the inspiration you need to know that you can do it too. These women are nothing short of inspiring and many of them didn't start exercising until later in life, so it is definitely possible to become fit even if you get a late start.

Lauren Piskin

Age: 53

The former competitive figure skater works out around 5 times a week mainly teaching classes at her two fitness studios.

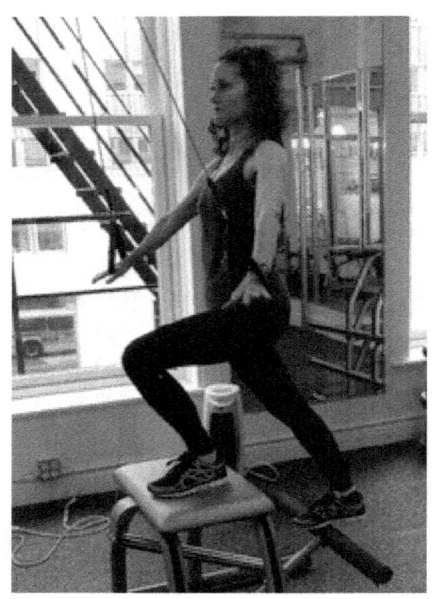

Elisabeth Halfpapp

Age: 56

Halfpapp credits yoga, core fusion and ballet six times per week with her healthy and fit. She also eats lots of leafy greens, sleep, positivity and her happy marriage for helping her stay healthy.

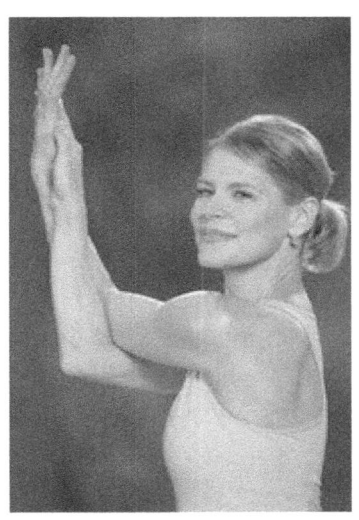

Ernestine Shepherd

She is currently 79 years old if you can believe it! She was listed by the Guinness Book of World Records as the oldest competitive female bodybuilder in 2010 and 2011. She has run nine marathons and teaches exercise classes for seniors and works as a personal trainer.

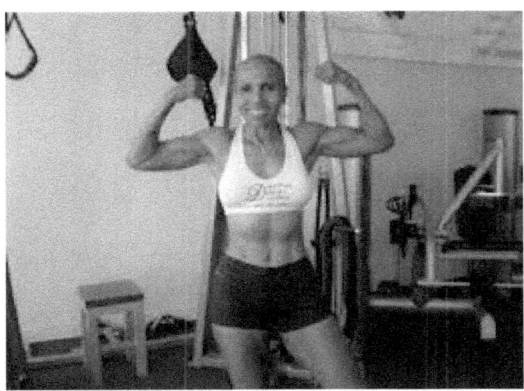

Bonus

Dinner meal plan for a week

Garlic Parmesan Chicken with Roasted Vegetables

- 2 garlic cloves, minced

- 2 tablespoons grated Parmesan cheese

- 3 teaspoons olive oil, divided

- 1 3 - ounce chicken breast

- 3 cups chopped vegetables (broccoli, potato, bell pepper)

- Salt and pepper to taste

  Preheat oven to 400 F. Mix together garlic, cheese and 1 tsp. oil. Pat garlic-cheese mixture onto chicken and place on baking sheet. Toss vegetables with 2 tsp. oil, salt and pepper and place on baking sheet. Cook for 20 minutes, or until chicken reaches 165 F and vegetables are tender.

Lemon Butter Salmon & Broccoli Penne

- 4 ounces salmon

- 3 ounces dry whole-grain penne pasta

- 1 1/2 cups frozen broccoli florets

- 1 tablespoon butter, melted

- 4 tablespoons low-sodium vegetable broth or water

- 1 lemon, zested and juiced

- 1 garlic clove, minced

Broil in a foil-lined broiler pan or grill salmon for about 8 minutes per inch of thickness. Cook pasta according to package directions. Heat broccoli in microwave until warm, about 4 minutes. Whisk together melted butter, broth or water, lemon zest and juice, and garlic. Toss penne with broccoli and place cooked salmon on top. Drizzle lemon-butter sauce over all.

Pinto Bean Tacos

- 1/2 cup canned pinto beans, rinsed and drained
- 1 lime, juiced
- 1/4 teaspoon cumin
- 1/4 teaspoon chili powder
- 2 whole-grain tortillas
- 1 cup shredded romaine lettuce
- 1/2 cup chopped tomato
- 1/4 avocado, chopped

In a microwave-safe bowl, warm beans, lime juice, cumin and chili powder. Put bean mixture into tortillas and top with lettuce, tomatoes and avocado.

BBQ Chicken Sandwich with Spinach Salad

- 2 tablespoons barbecue sauce
- 1 3 - ounce chicken breast (or use rotisserie chicken, skin removed)
- 2 cups baby spinach
- 1/2 cup shredded carrots
- 2 tablespoons slivered walnuts
- 2 tablespoons balsamic vinaigrette
- 1 whole-grain hamburger bun, toasted

Brush barbecue sauce on chicken and bake or grill in foil until it reaches 165 F. (To save time, use rotisserie chicken, skin removed.) Toss spinach, carrots and walnuts with dressing. Put chicken on toasted bun; serve with salad.

Steak Salad with Lemon Walnut Vinaigrette & Whole Grain Roll

- 3 ounces steak

- 1 lemon, juiced

- 1 tablespoon olive oil

- 2 tablespoons walnuts

- 1 teaspoon Dijon mustard

- 3 cups baby spinach

- 1 whole-grain roll

- Grill or broil steak until it reaches about 160 F (medium), and slice. In a blender or mini food processor, pulse lemon juice, oil, walnuts and mustard until smooth. Toss spinach and steak slices with dressing.
- Serve with whole-grain roll.

Fried Rice Bowl with Broccoli and Shrimp

- 2 garlic cloves, minced

- 1 tablespoon peanut oil

- 1 1/2 cups chopped broccoli

- 1 cup cooked brown rice (use precooked, microwavable or frozen)

- 3 ounces (about 12 large) frozen cooked shrimp, thawed

- 2 tablespoons chopped peanuts

Sauté garlic in oil for 2 minutes. Add broccoli and cook for 8 minutes, or until tender. Add cooked rice and thawed shrimp to pan; warm for 3 to 4 minutes. Top with peanuts.

Spinach and Goat Cheese Flatbread Pizza

- 2 whole-grain flatbreads

- 1/2 cup pizza sauce

- 2 tablespoons dried oregano

- 1 cup baby spinach

- 1/4 cup goat cheese

- 2 tablespoons pine nuts

Preheat oven to 350 F. Bake flatbread for 7 minutes. Spread pizza sauce on flatbread and top with oregano, spinach, goat cheese and pine nuts. Bake an additional 12 to 15 minutes.

For more information on diet and fitness over age 50 please visit:

Lindamelone.com

Fitandfabliving.cim

Fitnessmagazine.com

Wellandgood.com

Nextavenue.org

Huffingtonpost

Aarp.com

Bodybuilding.com

Boomerbrief.com

Conclusion

I want to thank and congratulate you on finishing this book. You are on your way to a great new life that is well within your reach. You have exactly what it takes to reach your fitness and weight loss goals, at 50, 60, 70 and beyond. As you can see from the women above, age in only a number and you can reach your fitness goals at any age. Age is not a factor that limits us, we are the only thing that can limit us.

I wish you nothing but health, wealth and wellness for you future.

Thank you again for downloading this book, I hope it helped you.

All the best,

Faith

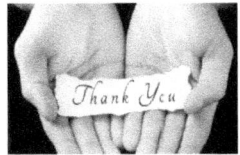

Finally, if you enjoyed this book, then I'd like to ask you for a favor, would you be kind enough to leave a review for this book on Amazon? It'd be greatly appreciated!

Thank you and good luck!

Preview of 'No Diet Weight Loss: The Simple No BS Plan to Lose Weight Without the Struggle'

The first step to long lasting and lifelong health and weight maintenance is to investigate and discover your trigger (s). Your trigger is in essence something that triggers you to overeat, or make poor food choices. Our triggers are usually start in childhood, when we learn to associate food with comfort. A crying baby is given a bottle to soothe him. If you fall and skin your arm, you might get a cookie or ice cream as a treat to feel better. Most of us are trained from a young age to associate tasty food with comfort and relief. Maybe it's your stressful job, maybe it's your family situation, and maybe it's a past trauma that you are trying to numb yourself into forgetting or comfort yourself with food to feel better about. It could be any number of things, but whatever it is, you need to identify it. It could also be physical issue such as a bad back, bad knees or a slow metabolism. The sooner you can identify what is causing you to overeat and/or not exercise as you should, the better. It's the only way to create a long lasting solution.

As I said, for me I was a stress eater, I would eat whenever I was anxious or there was a lot going on in my life. I realized that I could no longer use food as a crutch for my stress. It wasn't healthy for me, and it left me feeling terrible afterwards. In order to deal with your triggers, identify what they are, and then the next step is to find a substitute to replace your trigger.

For me, I found it effective to meditate, or workout when I was feeling overly stressed. Afterwards I feel relaxed and am no longer dependent upon food as my crutch. Below you will find a few suggestions for stress relievers if you too are a stress eater like myself:

Stress relief activities

Write/journal your feelings

Talk to a friend

Play with your pet

Listen to music

Get a massage

Work on a craft project

Go for a walk

Limit internet/cell phone use

Drink some hot tea

Laugh-watch a funny show/movie

Take a hot bath

Deep breathing

These methods have been proven to help reduce stress and anxiety and I definitely integrate them into my relaxation routine. I love getting into a hot bath and relaxing away the stress of the day. Just find what works for you, and go with it. If there's something that's not listed that helps you relax, absolutely just do it!

I know some people don't have a specific trigger that makes you overeat, but you are somehow still overweight. Well, if your issue is a physical one, for example a bad knee, or bad back, once you identify what the problem is, you can figure out how to circumvent it. For example, your doctor can tell you what exercises you can safely do in order to workout without further injuring your knee. If you have a very slow metabolism, there are certain techniques as well as certain foods that are known to naturally boost your metabolism and help you maintain a healthy weight.

Chapter 3

Metabolism and You

**Metabolism boosting foods:

Blueberries- 'Antioxidant' seems to be the new buzzword of this decade. Everyone needs more antioxidants. Everyone wants more antioxidants. Everyone buys foods with antioxidants; but do we know what they are?

Oxidation is a chemical process within your body whereby electrons are taken off a substance via a chemical reaction. When your body undergoes oxidative stress, such as when you're sick, have a disease or after a workout, the product from this oxidation is known as a 'free radical'.

When free radicals start to build up in your body because they're not cleared, they start to damage cells which can lead to inhibited muscle growth, fat loss or even cause disease. Good thing we have antioxidants like blueberries. Antioxidants help prevent this oxidation from taking place, and thus prevents the buildup of free radicals.

Almonds- Almonds are truly one of nature's miracle foods. You get such a big bang for your buck. First of all, almonds are nutritionally dense. This means that for a small portion size, you get a large amount of healthy macronutrients and calories (but GOOD calories).

Independent studies have shown that almonds are the most nutritionally dense nut; so almonds provide the most healthy calories and nutrition for the smallest serving size. You get the most nutrition possible out of the calories you eat.

One serving of almonds, or about a handful, is an excellent source of vitamin E (an antioxidant) and a good source of fiber (which helps keep you full). Almonds also offer heart-healthy monounsaturated fat.

Nine clinical studies over the last thirteen years have shown that almonds can lower cholesterol as part of a diet low in saturated fat. These groundbreaking studies show how a handful of almonds a day consistently lowered LDL cholesterol levels. Eating almonds is a filling snack. Almonds contain protein, fiber and monounsaturated fat, all which may help keep you satisfied.

Whey protein- Whey protein (the highest quality and best form of protein) is amazing stuff. It provides the body with the necessary building blocks to produce amino acids that are used for building muscle tissue.

Nearly everyone who weight trains knows the importance of protein supplementation. Studies have been conducted that compare whey protein to other sources. They have found that whey protein contains the perfect combination of overall amino acid (the building blocks of protein) makeup, and in just the right concentrations for optimal performance in the body.

Both hormonal and cellular responses seem to be greatly enhanced with supplementation of whey protein as well. Not to mention the benefits whey protein has on the body's immune system.

Whey protein also plays a role as an antioxidant and helps support a healthy immune system. Most importantly, consistent whey protein intake coupled with exercise will result in consistent muscle building and potential fat loss.

Salmon- Although it's higher in calories than most whitefish, salmon is low in saturated fat, yet high in protein, and a unique type of healthy fat, the omega-3 essential fatty acid.

As their name implies, essential fatty acids are essential for human health but because they cannot be made by the body, they must be obtained from foods.

Fish contain a type of essential fatty acid called the omega-3 fatty acids. Fish like salmon are higher in omega-3 fatty acids than warm water fish. In addition to being an excellent source of omega-3s, salmon are an excellent source of selenium, and a very good source of protein, niacin and vitamin B12, and a good source of phosphorous, magnesium and vitamin B6.

The omega-3 fats found in salmon have a broad range of beneficial cardiovascular effects. Omega-3s help prevent erratic heart rhythms, make blood less likely to clot inside arteries (the prominent cause of heart attacks and strokes), improve the ratio of good cholesterol to bad cholesterol, and can help prevent the clogging of arteries.

Spinach- First and foremost, you'll get forearms like Popeye. Just joking. Leafy green vegetables like spinach with its delicate texture and jade green color provide more nutrients than any other food.

By eating spinach, you'll be protecting yourself against osteoporosis, heart disease, colon cancer, arthritis, and other diseases at the same time. And if the physical benefits aren't enough, you also get mental improvements.

In animal studies, researchers have found that spinach may help protect the brain from oxidative stress and may reduce the effects of age-related related declines in brain function. Researchers found that feeding aging laboratory animals spinach-rich diets significantly improved both their learning capacity and motor skills.

Turkey- Turkey is naturally low in fat without the skin, containing only 1 gram of fat per ounce of flesh. A 5-ounce serving provides almost half of the recommended daily allowance of folic acid, and is a good source of vitamins B, B1, B6, zinc and potassium.

These nutrients have been found to keep blood cholesterol down, protect against birth defects, cancer and heart disease, aid in nerve function and growth, boost the immune system, regulate blood pressure, and assist in healing processes.

Turkey is also extremely high in protein, which is great for build muscle and losing fat because it keeps the metabolism revving, and helps fuel the muscles before, during and after a workout.

Oatmeal- I'm not talking about the sugar-laden single-servings packages of instant oatmeal that come in a million different flavors. I'm talking about plain, boring, large, slow-cooking rolled oats. You could also do the quick oats as well, just make sure that whatever type you choose doesn't come with any added sugar.

Oats are a great source of both insoluble and soluble fiber. Insoluble fiber's cancer-fighting properties are due to the fact that it attacks certain bile acids, reducing their toxicity.

Soluble fiber may reduce LDL cholesterol without lowering HDL cholesterol. LDL is bad; HDL is good. Soluble fiber also slows down the digestion of starch. This may be beneficial to diabetics because, when you slow down the digestion of starch, you avoid the sharp rises in your blood sugar level (insulin spikes) that usually occur following a meal.

It has been found that those who eat more oats are less likely to develop heart disease, a disease that is currently widespread in the United States. The phytochemicals in oat may also have cancer-fighting properties. Oats are a good source of many nutrients including vitamin E, zinc, selenium, copper, iron, manganese and magnesium. Oats are also a good source of protein.

Check out my other books

Smoothies for Weight Loss: 100 Delicious Smoothie Recipes for Rapid Weight Loss, Detox and Increased Energy

Chronic Pain: The Ultimate Guide to Beat Chronic Pain and Regain Your Life

Rheumatoid Arthritis: Proven Strategies to Prevent and Reverse Arthritis Pain For Good

The Insomnia Solution: The Ultimate Guide to Cure Your Insomnia For Life